MW01671039

DARE TO CARE. ECOFEMINISM AS A SOURCE OF INSPIRATION

Dare to Care

Ecofeminism as a source of inspiration

GREEN EUROPEAN FOUNDATION

SKRIBIS

The Green European Foundation (GEF) is a European-level political foundation whose mission is to contribute to a lively European sphere of debate and to foster greater involvement by citizens in European politics. GEF strives to mainstream discussions on European policies and politics both within and beyond the Green political family. The foundation acts as a laboratory for new ideas, offers cross-border political education and a platform for cooperation and exchange at the European level.

Oikos is a Flemish think tank that strives for social-ecological change by contributing to public debate from an ecological perspective. Oikos focuses on long term challenges that are crucial for the future of our society and coming generations. Oikos wants to provide an inspiring framework for positive practices. In seminars, lectures, publications and opinion pieces, the different dimensions of this aspiration to change are deliberated: the underlying ethics, the analysis of the current situation and the development of alternatives, together with concrete strategies to get there.

This English-language edition is published by the Green European Foundation, with the support of Oikos and the financial support of the European Parliament. The views expressed are solely those of the authors and do not necessarily reflect the views of the European Parliament.

Contact the Green European Foundation:
Rue du Fossé 3, L-1536 Luxembourg
Brussels office: Mundo Madou, Avenue des Arts 7-8,
1210 Brussels, Belgium
Tel: +32 2 329 00 50
Email: info@gef.eu
Website: www.gef.eu

Copies of the book can be ordered
by sending an email request to info@gef.eu

Contents

Foreword to the English version

The COVID-19 pandemic has taught us a series of lessons. The first, obvious lesson is that each country separately is incapable of coping with such a massive emergency. When it comes to tackling international crises, the European Union has an important role to play. An adequate political response was and is only possible through cooperation at an international level.

More fundamentally however, the reality is that nature destruction – including massive deforestation in the "Global South" for the sake of our extractive economy – contributes directly to the spread of disease-causing zoonoses like COVID-19. The pandemic thus not only proved the importance of a high-performance healthcare infrastructure, but has also highlighted how crucial it is to take care of *more-than-human worlds*. This translates, among other things, into the need for an ambitious European biodiversity policy, embedded in the global biodiversity strategy.

Ultimately, the crux of our interconnected crises lies in the need for a different economic policy *tout court*.

As long as we continue to rely on the extraction of raw materials for production; as long as the European economy does not become a regenerative one, restoring and maintaining the biosphere, we will continue to run around in circles. This is made clear for instance in the illuminating report *Why the European Green Deal needs ecofeminism* (2021), that rightly observes: "the reliance on the healing powers of the so-called free market, that is set to be more efficient in managing public goods, fails to regard the interconnectedness of the economy, our society, and the environment".[1]

"While there is increasing consensus that we need to decarbonize our economies (exemplified by agreements of green deal packages such as the European Green Deal), transforming towards this conception of a "green economy" will not be enough to drastically reduce emissions, nor to enhance gender and social justice as it strongly relies on technological innovation, green investments and green consumerism, thus failing to include intersectional social justice".[2]

Recognizing this need for a more fundamental change, and based on conceptions of interconnection, equity and intersectionality, we introduce in this essay an economy of care. An economy that links environmentalism and sustainability to social justice, by emphasizing how the environment intersects with other social issues such as inequality, sexism and racism.[3]

Introduction

As we write this introduction, New York has suffered unprecedented flooding. Cars float around, the subway is knee-deep in water. In the space of one hour, more rain has fallen than ever recorded. South Sudan, Kenya, Niger and Chad have also been hit by serious floods in the past year. It chimes with what the Indian author Amitav Ghosh notes in his book *The Great Derangement: Climate Change and the Unthinkable* (2016). As coastal cities, Mumbai and New York are extremely susceptible to flooding and other natural disasters. This is no coincidence, but a direct consequence of the way they were conceived: from 'a colonial vision on the world, in which proximity to the water represents power and security, mastery and conquest.' That was not always so: many old port cities in Asia, as well as in Europe, are further inland and hence better protected. It is as if the need to consider 'the unpredictable furies of the ocean' was widely acknowledged in former times, Ghosh writes. But with the rise of the British Empire those insights were jettisoned and port cities built right by the sea. As a result, metropolises such as Jakarta are now at risk from the rise in sea level and will need to be relocated. Thinking that we can ignore nature as actor is a form of fatal hubris. That much was clear when a tsunami swept over Fukushima's nuclear power station.

Instead, we propose the power of an ethics of care based on the premise that as human beings we are part of the web of life and rooted in natural and social relationships and interdependencies. It is this myriad of connections that give humans their identity. The African proverb 'it takes a village to raise a child' encapsulates this idea well.

This alternative calls for changes to some of the fundamental assumptions of our society. This will only come about when the economy is once more embedded in the democratic values of an ethics of care. What we talk about, how we view the world and one another, the concrete actions we take: it is all interrelated. That means we need to reground ourselves and once again shoulder responsibility for the world we live in; view that world with an open mind and a sense for solidarity. This is not an individual, but a collective, political mission.

That brings us to the structure of this essay, which we approach as a thought experiment. In the first chapter, we will set out to introduce ecofeminism as an analytical framework and a source of inspiration that is both powerful and more pertinent than ever. In the second chapter we start our analysis with concrete historical context before we outline a new, hopeful perspective on how we might achieve a caring society and a genuine economy of care. We argue the case for placing care where it belongs: as one of the leading principles at the heart of a just society, which we should all endeavour to work towards.

This is not an easy task, that much is clear. It calls for a critical examination of some of the essential aspects of the dominant modern-western mode of being. We have, in fact, known for decades that we need to do this. At this juncture in time, when we have billionaires dreaming of travelling to Mars, it is astonishing to read what the Jewish-German philosopher Hannah Arendt tasked us with as early as 1958. In her book about the Human Condition, she notes that, in the first place, we must trace back 'modern world alienation, its twofold flight from the earth into the universe and from the world into the self, to its origins'.[4] Only by re-establishing equal relationships with everybody on Earth, recognising that we are part of more-than-human worlds and fostering those connections, will we be able to exercise the necessary care to ensure a liveable future, with a view to a good life for all. Because we want to take care of everyone.

CHAPTER 1

An ethics of care

It is summer. The European continent is seeing infernal temperatures in some regions and cataclysmic floods in others. Canada, Spain and Italy break temperature records, yet again, while fierce wildfires rage across Algeria and Morocco, claiming scores of casualties. In other parts of the world, huge migrant and refugee caravans cross deserts and seas, hoping to reach more habitable regions, and all too often perishing in the process. Amidst the more immediate impact on people's lives, it's easy to forget the damage to ecosystems and the long-term consequences for the future.

This is not the script of some scary sci-fi film: we are talking summer 2021. The coronavirus continues to hold humanity to ransom. Around the world, 'caring for one another' became a key point of focus when the COVID-19 pandemic first hit. Within the space of a year, nursing in many countries evolved from an understaffed and underappreciated profession to a hugely popular subject to study. Yet at the same time patents, towering vaccine prices and Big Pharma's hunger for profit are, in a cynical paradox, preventing the vaccination of billions of people. Life has ground to a halt in many areas. People are dying. Global solidarity is a distant proposition.

> 'What is this thing that has happened to us? It's a virus, yes. In and of itself it holds no moral brief. But it is definitely more than a virus. [...] Whatever it is, coronavirus has made the mighty kneel and brought the world to a halt like nothing else could. Our minds are still racing back and forth, longing for a return to "normality", trying to stitch our future to our past and refusing to acknowledge the rupture. But the rupture exists. And in the midst of this terrible despair, it offers us a chance to rethink the doomsday machine we have built for ourselves. Nothing could be worse than a return to normality. Historically, pandemics have forced humans to break with the past and imagine their world anew. This one is no different. It is a portal, a gateway between one world and the next. We can choose to walk through it, dragging the carcasses of our prejudice and hatred, our avarice, our data banks and dead ideas, our dead rivers and smoky skies behind us. Or we can walk through lightly, with little luggage, ready to imagine another world. And ready to fight for it.'
> — Arundhati Roy[5]

The system, as it is, is not working. It is a doomsday machine, marginalising too many people and causing too much damage to the world around us. We need a system change, a transformation of the economy and a reorganisation of society. The 2019 report by the IPBES (Intergovernmental Science-Policy Platform on Biodiversity and Ecosystem Services) stressed this need for transformative social change, which it defined as 'a fundamental reorganization of economic and social systems, including changes in paradigms and values.'[6] The findings of the most recent IPCC report confirm this: if we keep on our current course the rise in global temperatures will not be limited to 1.5°C, but increase to 2, 3 or even 4°C. The consequences will be catastrophic for both humans and the environment.

This does not only call for the transformation of existing structures so they work within the limits of our planet, we need a culture shift, too. Every system change starts with a change in mentality, a different world view. The American systems thinker Donella Meadows puts it aptly: 'The shared idea in the minds of society, the great big unstated assumption – unstated because unnecessary to state; everyone already knows them – constitute that society's paradigm, or deepest set of beliefs about how the world works.'[7] Today's socio-ecological crises originate in a number of dominant ideas in contemporary society: the notion that one person is superior to another and that humans are superior to all other life; that nature is a lifeless heap of raw materials, a mere backdrop to our lives; that economic growth is vital to our well-being so we have to keep producing and consuming.

Ecofeminism provides a framework for creating a break with our fundamental convictions. This essay seeks to acknowledge the inspiring thinkers who help bring about the constructive change that is so vitally important to future generations. Using ecology as a starting point while keeping in mind that everything on our planet is connected, we want to contribute to the political discourse needed to shape the necessary social changes. We are hoping to play a positive part in building a movement that is constantly evolving and that aims to make our world a beautiful, tolerant and good place to live. A place that will remain liveable for those after us, from the smallest fungus to the largest rainforest and all the people on our Earth.

1. The footsteps in which we follow

The French philosopher Emilie Hache dates the emergence of ecofeminism as a school of thought to the political context of the 1980s.[8] The publication of the Club of Rome report *The Limits to Growth* in 1972, the nuclear arms race during the Cold War, mass deforestation around the world and various famines marked the start of the global ecological crisis.[9]

Ecofeminism has its roots in the activism of that era. The French philosopher Françoise d'Eaubonne is widely credited with coining the term in 1974, although some authors argue that it cropped up in different places at the time.[10]

Confronted with the nuclear threat and the destruction of our habitat, various feminist collectives began taking coordinated action. Nuclear power stations were blockaded, roads barricaded and people took to the streets, chaining themselves to fences and trees. It was during those protests that the first texts with an ecofeminist slant were written.[11] These women discovered parallels between the way modern society treated the Earth and the way it treated people who differed from the white male norm. The natural environment was regarded as a reservoir of dead matter, ready for extraction. Women and people of colour were seen as inferior. It is at this juncture between the destruction of nature and social oppression that we find ecofeminism.

One of the major inspirations for ecofeminists worldwide was the Indian Chipko movement. This female-led movement emerged in the 1970s and became an international model for the protection of the environment and the future of the community.[12] In the Garhwal hills, an extensive and delicate ecosystem in the Indian Himalayas where the Ganges has its source, the forests were historically managed as communal resources with strict, albeit informal, social mechanisms for keeping its exploitation in check and the ecosystem balanced.[13] But in the early 1970s, the region was hit by devastating floods and earthquakes. Mass deforestation higher up and the replacement of the original deciduous trees by more profitable pines for commercial exploitation were found to have been the cause of these disasters.[14] The deciduous forest had played a central role in maintaining soil and water stability even after heavy rain, so its replacement by lucrative pines was ruinous.[15] The devastation was immense, the human suffering and damage to the natural world compounded by the significant economic impact on the local population.

The years that followed saw numerous protests against commercial forest exploitation. The very first Chipko action took place spontaneously in April 1973, with villagers demonstrating against the felling of ash trees in Mandal Forest.[16] In March 1974, twenty-seven women saved yet more trees from the 'contractor's axe'.[17] Their tactic was to spread around the forest and embrace the trees so they could not be cut. The Hindi word '*chipko*' literally means 'to stick', and it is in this form of nonviolent resistance, which goes back more than three hundred years in India, that the term 'tree hugger' has its origins.

By 1975, over three hundred villages in the region faced the ongoing threat of earthquakes caused by commercial exploitation. Increased erosion and the resulting decline in land productivity meant that villages that had been self-sufficient in the past now had to resort to importing food.[18] The protests widened. Today Chipko is a national movement, which has managed to force a fifteen-year ban on commercial logging in the region and to block clearcutting in the Western Ghats and the Vindhya Range. It also continues to press for a nation-wide forest policy that is more responsive to people's needs and the land's ecological requirements.[19]

Ecofeminism is first and foremost a political framework,[20] a lens through which to look critically at the world, exploring 'the interconnections of dominance between humans and between humans and the earth'.[21] It is a perspective that clearly shows that environmental destruction and social oppression have the same origin. One of the main themes running through this body of thought is the question of care for the community. What are the social, biological and emotional conditions for looking after, repairing and healing damaged communities and environments?[22] An ethics of care focuses on the inextricable link between human and non-human nature and on 'affective engagement' with the world around us.[23] Seeing the compound, interconnected socio-ecological crises, ecofeminists around the globe point to the importance of a caring commitment and dedication that are currently lacking in public discourse.[24] 'The resilience of ecosystems, unpaid and unrecognized forms of work, social reciprocity and care are unvalued or undervalued.'[25] This has been a factor in 'the dispossession of peoples from their land and livelihood, the destruction of natural habitat and the general degradation of the environment'.[26] Ecofeminism seeks to facilitate the transition from 'unhealthy, life-denying systems and relationships to healthy, life-affirming ones'.[27] We need to evolve towards a new enchantment with the world, and rethink the place of human beings in it. We need a new logic, one that views each person as part of a web of relationships, that ties individual wellbeing to the flourishing of others and considers the importance of healthy relationships and context.[28]

A fully integrative project, ecofeminism seeks to develop an alternative to our present culture.[29] This fits in with what Vandana Shiva and Maria Mies have termed the ecological shift:[30]

> 'The ecological shift involves not seeing ourselves as outside the ecological web of life, as masters, conquerors and owners of the earth's resources. It means seeing ourselves as members of the earth family, with responsibility to care for other species and life on earth in all its diversity, from the tiniest microbe to the largest mammal. It creates the imperative to live, produce and consume within ecological limits and within our share of ecological space, without encroaching on the rights of other species and other people.'

2. 'We are as Gods and we had better get used to it'[31]

Where do our prevailing western notions about the world come from? Why is it that we are incapable of taking a balanced approach to our living environment?

Many historians and philosophers of science point to the Enlightenment and the advance of modern science as the period in which people began to atomise, objectify and dissect nature. In doing so, we evolved from an organic worldview to a mechanical one. In her book *The Death of Nature: Women, Ecology and the Scientific Revolution* (1980), ecofeminist and historian of science Carolyn Merchant shows that the rise of industry in the seventeenth century made new technologies such as windmills and cranes an important part of everyday life. Western thinkers began to impose a mechanical order on the world, seeing organisms as entities that could be taken apart, like a clock. The emphasis now shifted to experimental science, with physics taking the lead. And while scientists such as Isaac Newton conceded that it was God who created nature, they also demonstrated that man can discover the laws of this nature.[32]

The impact on western philosophy was immense: by the end of the seventeenth century our understanding of the cosmos was changing. The era saw a shift in our image of humans and the world: the original conception of nature as a living organism (the organic cosmos) evolved to the belief that nature functions like a machine (the mechanical cosmos). Western man began to see nature as a reservoir of dead matter that he could analyse, use and manipulate as he pleased. And as other peoples were perceived as primitive and inferior, this 'faith in progress' had to be imposed on them too.

The influential French philosopher René Descartes believed that the key to power over nature lay in the fact that matter can be divided into constituent parts. The resulting data could then be manipulated according to a set of mathematical rules and models. The 'death of the world soul' and the 'removal of nature's spirits', which took away 'any scruples that might be associated with the view that nature was a living organism', resulted in the increasing destruction of the environment.[33] Machines came to symbolise the order of life itself. Serving as models for western philosophy and science, they held the promise of power and domination over nature. In other words, modern science offered a way of consolidating man's control over nature. Some of the convictions that Merchant believes were conducive to this are:[34]

- nature consists of dead, inert and passive components;
- nature is full of patterns, which is why the scientific domain can be reduced to rules, regulations and laws;

- the world can be predicted, described and controlled by science, just like a machine can be controlled by man.

The legacy of enlightenment thinking persists to this day and determines our dominant worldview. This is reflected in, among other things, the way governments and industry try to solve the climate crisis:[35] they are hoping that by throwing more innovation and more technology at the problem they can fix both the earth and the climate, as though they were a machine and its thermostat. The underlying structures, the growth mindset and increasing inequality are never questioned, let alone tackled.

In the economic sphere these ideas took shape in the theories of Adam Smith and the invisible hand of the market. His reasoning can be summarised as follows: people are like atoms, competitive and only interested in their own wellbeing. But the community actually benefits from this self-interest. The baker bakes bread to sell and survives by exchanging the fruits of his labour for money. While he may be looking after his own interest, we get to buy the bread and obtain food. In this way the baker indirectly contributes to the welfare of the community.[36] However, journalist Katrine Marçal is clear when she asserts:[37]

> 'For the butcher, the baker and the brewer to be able to go to work, at the time Adam Smith was writing, their wives, mothers or sisters had

> to spend hour after hour, day after day minding the children, cleaning the house, cooking the food, washing the clothes, drying tears and squabbling with the neighbours. However you look at the market, it is always built on another economy. An economy that we rarely discuss.'

Another profound impact of enlightenment thinking on our worldview was the emergence of an artificial divide between nature and culture, making the idea that nature is separate from man a relatively recent invention. Ever since, the world has been structured around these two dimensions, with one, culture, superior to the other, nature. On one side of the dichotomy you had the superior ratio, the mind, culture, transcendence, science and the masculine. On the other side inferior matter, the emotional, physical, caring, natural, the feminine. This artificial divide has had an enormous impact on the way we organise our society to this day. Binary thought has embedded itself in our minds and has been passed, subconsciously, from generation to generation. There is, for example, no such thing as a 'domestic gene', which, for biological reasons, would assign the task of ironing to women.[38] Yet we continue to see care and domestic responsibilities as 'feminine', even in the twenty-first century.[39] Household chores form the background that facilitates 'the real work', the work of men. Non-human nature is viewed in the same way: it is still seen as the backdrop against which human life unfolds.

3. The story of the master and the slave

The Australian philosopher and ecofeminist Val Plumwood has given a powerful account of this binary thinking in her work *Feminism and the Mastery of Nature* (1997). Plumwood believes that we are unable to acknowledge our dependence on ecological processes because our western rationality places human identity outside nature. Cartesian thought, Plumwood argues, has created a gulf between 'conscious' humanity and 'mindless' nature. This leads us to view environmental problems as somehow separate from us, to think that climate change will not affect us. However, we are just as dependent on a healthy biosphere as other forms of life.

Not only did rational thought place man outside nature and thereby create a dichotomy between nature and culture, it also brought about other dualisms: reason versus emotion, man versus woman, master versus slave, with one superior to the other. It is the latter dualism that can serve as a model for understanding the world today, according to Plumwood. Contrary to some feminists' claims, she believes it is not masculinity in and of itself that is problematic, but the cultural identity of the master in relation to the slave, within the contexts of class, gender, sex and nature. Plumwood labels this the dominator identity. When it spreads among populations through culture and science, people will start to behave accordingly. In Plumwood's words: 'The *material* and the *cultural spheres* both do *the work of domination*.'[40] Social domination, exclusion and hierarchy then come to be seen as inevitable, as part of human nature. This ends up distorting perception on either side: that of both master and slave, both coloniser and colonised.

The crux of the problem can therefore be traced back to the development of hierarchical and binary thought, which casts everything in terms of higher or lower, more or less intelligent, better or worse. These artificial constructs legitimise the oppression of the other (that is to say, everybody who is not included in the cultural category of the western, 'rational', white male). Power and exclusion are institutionalised.

Plumwood stresses that a dualism is not the same as a difference or a contrast. In a dualistic structure, as in a hierarchy, the culture and values associated with the other are systematically portrayed as inferior. Hierarchies are theoretically open to change, but once they are entrenched in the culture, any change becomes difficult. Plumwood has identified five different mechanisms[41] that enable and reproduce this dualistic worldview.

To begin with, there is backgrounding. This mechanism sees us benefiting from the other's services, without acknowledging them, before going on to minimise the importance of those services or contributions. Think of the attention to and respect for management roles ('manager of the year'), whereas there would not even be a managing position without the employees that do the actual work. One person serves as the background to the 'real' work of the other. Another example: the fundamental work carried out daily by stay-at-home mothers, which enables the father to do the 'real' job, outside the home. In fact, even when the woman does enter the job market, she will still provide most of the care within the family. That makes the number of women working part-time four times higher than men in our society. And part-time work means a lower wage, followed by a lower pension later.[42] A further example of backgrounding is nature serving as a décor for the 'real' action, with humans in the leading role. But it is the master who needs the slave more than the other way around.

Secondly, polarisation is the basis for radical exclusion. The difference between two groups or two people can be magnified and emphasised to such a degree that the other appears to be from a different world altogether. At the same time, all possible similarities are erased and minimised and anything bridging the two ignored. Extreme right-wing or nationalist political parties tend to deploy this tactic, which depicts the differences between groups of people as unbridgeable.

Thirdly, every other is incorporated in the dominant culture, forced to assimilate and adapt. As Simone de Beauvoir said: 'Humanity is male and man defines woman ... as relative to him.'[43] In this mindset, one's own position is the centre to which all others relate. What's more, the others are only seen as 'good' when they adapt fully to the dominant group. Think of the myth of good immigrants, in which newcomers who speak foreign tongues will only be well received by the culture of destination if they are grateful and obliging, 'integrate' perfectly, speak the language fluently and refrain from as many native customs as possible.

The fourth mechanism Plumwood identifies is instrumentalism: the master's purposes are imposed on the slave, and the slave is used as a means to an end. Even though the master-slave relationship is presented as being in the interest of both parties, it is abundantly clear that the slave draws the short straw. This is reflected in the identity of this group and the qualities expected of them: the dutiful housewife, the quiet, diligent worker, the grateful colonised people.

Finally, Plumwood introduces the concept of homogenisation: by failing to acknowledge the diversity within the subordinate group, this demographic is made to look like a homogenous mass. And so we end up with monocultures not just in nature, but in the mind too.[44] Homogenisation reduces originally complex and diverse people and cultures to a uniform group, and in doing so consolidates stereotypes.

4. Intersectionality

> 'Feminism, as a liberation struggle, must exist apart from and as part of the larger struggle to eradicate domination in all its forms. We must understand that patriarchal domination shares an ideological foundation with racism and other forms of group oppression, that there is no hope that it can be eradicated while these systems remain intact.' – bell hooks[45]

To better understand how we can counter the cultural trend of dualism, we will take a more detailed look at intersectionality. The intersectional framework,* which is closely aligned with ecofeminism, helps us broaden our perspective and be sensitive to other identities and experiences, while showing respect for the differences between them. For example: whereas feminism champions women's rights and gender equality, intersectional feminism provides an insight

* Intersectionality exposes the convergence of various forms of exclusion and the dynamic that drives it. This inclusive perspective helps formulate more comprehensive solutions that consider the many different factors that determine our positions in society (source: Arikoglu *et al.*, 2014).

into the way women's overlapping identities – encompassing race, class, ethnicity, religion and sexual orientation – shapes their experience of oppression and discrimination.

This is where most definitions of intersectionality end, thereby missing the main reason Kimberlé Crenshaw coined the term: intersectionality addresses not only a person's various overlapping identities, but also how these identities interact with existing structures.[46] In the context of this essay the question then becomes: what impact does climate change have on the members of a marginalised group? Lawyer and researcher Daphina Misiedjan explains it with the help of an analogy:

> 'Picture the big environmental issues such as climate change and pollution like a big storm. We are all in it together, but the boats we are in are different. Some find themselves on a nice cruise ship, others on a small motorboat, while yet others have to make do with a raft or even less. The way in which the storm affects us varies. Some have the necessary means to protect themselves, others do not. How do we deal with this when everybody, also in times of climate change and pollution, has a right to a healthy life?'[47]

An intersectional lens allows us to decentre the dominant culture's narratives about certain subjects – in this case the climate crisis and the solutions that are being put forward – and make room for positions and perspectives that rarely get a look in but that are crucial for analysing *and* solving the problems. This is where intersectional thought and the idea of ecological justice meet, paving the way for a fairer approach to the problem as it now stands. The multifaceted framework needed to properly tackle the many ills of climate change calls for solutions for us all and not just for the happy few. In order to achieve this, we must understand how our many identities interact with existing structures.

Crenshaw (1989) sees intersectionality as a way of thinking about our identity and our relationship to power. Initially conceived to look at the position of black women in society, the term was soon found to apply to the many people from marginalised groups who are notionally part of society yet not really represented. Crenshaw: 'If you don't have a lens that's been trained to look at how various forms of discrimination come together, you're unlikely to develop a set of policies that will be as inclusive as they need to be.'[48] Ecofeminism builds on this by saying that humanity's 'freedom' depends not only on the freedom of nature and of women, but also on achieving that freedom for everybody on these fault lines.

The idea that the exploitation of the Earth and its resources is linked to the subjugation and oppression of women is not new. It posits that our relationship with the planet and its riches is historically intertwined with the dominant society's relationship with the female gender. In *The Nature of Race. Discourses of Racial Difference in Ecofeminism* (1997), Noël Sturgeon defines ecofeminism as 'a contemporary political movement operating on the theory that the ideologies which authorize injustices based on gender, race and class are related to the ideologies which sanction the exploitation and degradation of the environment'.[49] As a child of third-wave feminism, ecofeminism has historically made the connection between gender, race and the destruction of the environment, but now the time has come to incorporate intersectionality into the movement. With the help of new discourses about care, responsibility and justice, we can introduce a breath of fresh air into the various ways in which humanity relates to nature.

5. Ecowomanism

So why the need for ecowomanism? To understand the approach, let us begin by looking at womanism. In 1979 writer, poet and activist Alice Walker first used the term womanist in her short story 'Coming Apart', and again later in the essay collection *In Search of our Mother's Gardens: Womanist Prose* (1983). In it she defined a womanist as a black feminist or a feminist of colour. 'Womanist,' she writes, 'is to feminist as purple is to lavender.'[50]

You might wonder why Alice Walker thought it necessary to coin the term womanist, especially in relation to feminist. The fact is, feminism has historically barely accommodated women of colour, who have consequently had to create their own space within the feminist movement and develop theories outside the existing frameworks. It made black feminist theory a useful instrument for ordinary women to map out different forms of oppression. It did what mainstream feminism did not do: it looked specifically at the relationship between black women and women of colour and the various forms of (class, race and sexist) oppression they encountered.

Black feminism posits that the experience of black women cannot and must not be understood through the lens of either blackness or womanhood, but through both. Ever since the time of slavery, black women have been at the vanguard of the fight for emancipation. Yet their efforts have rarely been acknowledged. This trend continues to this day. Just think of the Ugandan Vanessa Nakate being cropped from a photo with other prominent climate activists Greta Thunberg, Loukina Tille, Luisa Neubauer and Isabelle Axelsson. As noted earlier, it is vitally important to understand the many expressions of the march to freedom, as the lessons we learn from each act of exclusion will lead to better, fairer solutions to the problems that afflict us today. The main one being the climate emergency.

In 'Challenging Patriarchal Structures: Wangari Maathai and the Green Belt Movement in Kenya,' Janet Muthuki (2006) analyses the Kenyan movement working on a green belt of trees, vegetation and fertile soil to combat deforestation and erosion and so safeguard the livelihoods of millions of people. Muthuki describes the Green Belt Movement as an example of African ecofeminist activism because of the way it tackles environmental issues, highlights gender relations and challenges patriarchal structures within the African context.

According to Melanie Harris, ecowomanism focuses on the perspectives of women of African heritage and reflects on the activist methods, religious practices and theories about tackling ecological injustice.[51] An ecowomanist approach is necessary because it stresses the link between social and ecological justice by recognising the overlapping and intersecting forms of oppression between women of colour and the environment.

It is also a useful term for conceptualising the paradoxical and problematic connections between women of colour and the Earth. As Harris puts it: 'In addition to honoring the beautiful connection that black women have with the earth, as the earth (earthlings) and as *shared creators,* black women have a particular historical experience of suffering with and as the earth.'[52] It is a reference to the transnational history of colonialism and slavery, which saw black women's bodies raped, objectified and sold for profit. Harris' take on the 'beautiful connection' between the bodies of black women and the Earth can be read as a romanticisation of knowledge systems, which couples the femininity of black women to a kind of primeval Earth wisdom and talks in ambivalent tones about both the positive and problematic links between the bodies of women of colour and the environment. As a result of this ambivalence, the idea of the female body can be used positively within ecological-activist representation, whereas the actual people may suffer physical and epistemic violence from outside forces.

The stories we tell here examine the relationship between humanity and the Earth, and the key role of humans in creating and maintaining responsible ecological practices. As discussed above, many ecology-centred theories still fail to adequately consider the racial, sexual and class-based oppression affecting many sections of society. Gendered ecologies on the other hand – whether they are referred to as African ecological activism or even as ecowomanism – prioritise race and gender as well as environmental awareness. They offer a lens through which to concentrate on women, children and families of colour, with a particular focus on the emancipation of an entire people.[53]

6. Indigenous cosmologies

In many First Nations*, the provision of basic needs and security as well as matters of spirituality are a collective responsibility. Edgar Villanueva beautifully illustrates this way of thinking in his book *Decolonising Wealth* (2021) in which he cites Dana Arviso, director of the Potlatch Fund and member of the Navajo:

> 'They told me they don't have a *word* for *poverty*. The closest thing that they had as an explanation for poverty was "to be *without family". They were saying it was a foreign concept to them that someone could be just so isolated and so without any sort of safety net or a family or a sense of kinship that they would be suffering from poverty*.'[54]

The ability to feed a community, to provide food for all, to live in balance with the land and to minimise internal and external conflicts is anchored in the First Nations way of life and passed on from one generation to the next. Because knowledge can disappear as people die, each generation sees it as their responsibility to preserve the culture by building on the community's wisdom and to pass the ancestral knowl-

* A term used to refer to North America's indigenous peoples.

edge on to children and grandchildren. First Nations often think about their actions in terms of the impact they will have on the seven generations after them. Under this so-called 'seven generation stewardship' what someone does is informed by the experience of the past seven generations, while it must also consider the seven to come: they, too, must benefit from these actions. Many First Nations have developed both formal rituals and informal training for the transfer of wisdom from the old to the young to ensure that the community can foster both personal and collective growth for all eternity.

Another example of community-rooted humanism is the African tradition of Ubuntu, which is short for the Zulu '*umuntu ngumuntu ngabantu*' and literally means that a person is a person through other persons. I am because you are. Asked what Ubuntu is, the South African archbishop and Nobel Peace Prize laureate Desmond Tutu replied: 'The profound truth is you cannot be human on your own. (...) We are human only through relationships. (...) We are really made for the delicate network of interdependence. (...) We are made for complementarity.'[55]

By offering compelling alternatives, indigenous knowledge systems pose a challenge to the status quo and constitute one of the paths to a fairer society for all. As value systems that have evolved and become embedded over time, they form an inspirational mirror that can teach us a great deal.

7. In nature's economy the currency is not money, it is life[56]

To the Indian scientist and ecofeminist Vandana Shiva it is clear: the destructive Anthropocene is not the only future; a paradigm shift is possible. You can see it happening all over the world, a change in consciousness is under way:

> 'It means shifting to *a focus on planetary and human* well-being, to living economies, to living well, to not having more, to valuing cooperation rather than competitiveness. These are the shifts being made by indigenous communities, peasants, women and young women in new movements.'[57]

These shifts involve working *with* the Earth, drawing on our intelligence to preserve and heal rather than conquer and wound. Shiva continues:

> 'For humans to protect life on Earth and their own future we need to become deeply conscious of the rights of Mother Earth [...] We need to get grounded again – in the Earth, her diversity, and her living processes – and unleash the positive forces of a creative Anthropocene. We will either make peace with the Earth or face extinction as humans [...] Continuing the war against the Earth is not an intelligent option.'[58]

This is first and foremost a cultural mission, as Amitav Ghosh argues in *The Great Derangement. Climate Change and the Unthinkable* (2016). Our inability, thus far, to tackle climate breakdown is primarily a crisis of the imagination. We are in need of other stories and fundamental beliefs, which may point us to a world in which we satisfy our basic needs in a way that helps protect and preserve the living environment of others. We need to imagine that everything can and must be different. An openness to other perspectives, experiences and ideas and a willingness to learn from other cultures and communities are crucial to this. We must be prepared to see what is thought of as normal as inconceivable instead, and to see the inconceivable that is taking place, such as climate breakdown, inequality and exploitation, for what it is. This receptivity will enable us to imagine, outside all existing frameworks, new representations of the good life that can turn our current reality into a liveable future.

CHAPTER 2

We all have our cares

1. Did we learn anything from the Covid pandemic?

It is something we read in all kinds of analyses: the coronavirus crisis helped us rediscover the importance of care. Remember, during the first lockdown, the applause for healthcare workers, who were forced to work too hard under precarious circumstances? And did it not teach us how vital it is to look after nature, because the felling of tropical forests directly contributes to the emergence of diseases such as COVID-19 and Ebola?

By now, we have long since stopped clapping, and the trees are still being cut. The real lesson is that caring is extremely difficult in an environment that is hostile to care. Society does not become more caring thanks to plenty of good will or because we are, in fact, 'humankind'.[59] For this to happen, changes to social structures and the underlying mindset are essential.

Besides, we quite carelessly accept how predatory capitalism is leading to one of the greatest health crises of the century: because we prioritise the appropriation and privatisation of knowledge via patents over and above care for our fellow human beings, billions of people in the Global South are denied the necessary coronavirus jabs. And this while the vaccines were largely developed with public money. But as the lockdowns have shown, our leaders find it more difficult to curtail property rights than to suspend our fundamental rights. Think of the introduction of a curfew or the violation of the right to education.

The world will not change merely in response to a theoretical exposition of an ethics of care, that much is clear. But it is a crucial first step. We can only turn the tide by looking at how an ethics of care can structurally underpin a caring society and an economy of care, and by acting accordingly. Caring calls for concrete action, for making a commitment. This potential for connection is tied to how we view the world and describe our *way of being*.

2. A world shaped by our words and views

When the British landed on the Australian coast in 1770, they saw that the area was already inhabited by people – the Aboriginals had in fact lived there for the past 50,000 years. But the Europeans, who believed themselves to be superior, viewed them as barbarians who did not have written laws and who did not make 'good' use of the land because they did not practise agriculture. This mattered, because Enlightenment thinker John Locke had argued that when people start cultivating land they can legitimately claim ownership of it. And because the Australian land mass was so dry and immense, the thinking went, it had to be virtually uninhabited. It was this reasoning that effectively underpinned the colonial myth. It allowed the newcomers to view the colossal island as *terra nullius*, or no man's land, which the coloniser could appropriate.

This is not purely ancient history. The old patterns of thinking and acting and the corresponding power relations have a lasting effect. It was not until 1992, after a legal case brought by a group of indigenous people, that the Australian Supreme Court ruled that the *terra nullius* doctrine had been unlawfully applied at the time.

Our words, our outlook and the corresponding assumptions shape how we treat the world. Later on, we illustrate this with reference to the research of Canadian forest ecologist Suzanne Simard. She experienced just how difficult it is to challenge entrenched ideas – in her case in forestry. It is no coincidence that after decades of ground-breaking research, she makes a passionate plea for replacing our reductionist science with complex systems thinking.

Systems thinking is based on the premise that everything is connected and interrelated. One of its architects is the American Donella Meadows, co-author of the Club of Rome's report, which we referred to at the start of this essay. *The Limits to Growth* was the first attempt at using systems thinking to analyse the interrelationships of major global phenomena, including population growth, industrialisation and the depletion of natural resources.

But what interests us here is the surprising insight that Meadows formulates in an essay in which she reflects on what she learned during her long and rich career.[60] When we want to achieve a system change – in our case a society based on an ethics of care – we tend to look at leverage points with puny effects. The use of subsidies is a good example. Subsidies to stimulate employees to work less only have a limited impact; the system itself remains largely the same. A redesign, which might include structurally shortening the working week for everybody, will have a bigger impact. But the leverage point with the greatest potential for change is the mindset of people, the prevailing social paradigm.

Meadows describes this fundamental issue very well when she says: 'In fact, we don't *talk about what we see*; we see only what we can talk about.' Those who think that nature and society evolve through competition will find examples of precisely that. But as soon as we have a different conversation and we seek out forms of cooperation and interdependence, we start discovering those positive principles everywhere. When we look at forestry, for instance, do we talk about a forest as a collection of trees in competition with one another, or as a complex, rich and vulnerable ecosystem?

3. When we can't see the wood for the trees

Born into a lumberjack family, Suzanne Simard took it for granted: humans need wood and take it from the forest. Her grandfather and uncles did so with great expertise: using horses, they would carefully remove a limited number of felled trees so the forest remained 'intact', and sell them to make a living. But as a teenager, Simard saw profit-seeking companies resorting more and more often to clearcutting, removing all the trees. They would then plant a monoculture of new trees on the resulting wasteland. But that was not all: when she found a job with a commercial logging business, the official line was that when planting new trees on such a clearcut, 'good practice' demanded the spraying of Roundup, the Monsanto herbicide, to eradicate all other life on the site. The argument was that any other plants or trees would run off with the light and nutrients. It is the capitalist take on what Darwin termed the survival of the fittest: evolution is based on the principles of competition and conflict. Simard soon observed that something about that reasoning was not right. Many of the newly planted Douglas firs died after the removal of the birches and aspen growing nearby. The removal of supposed rivals gave the survivors both more light and more room, and yet they did worse rather than better…

After obtaining a doctorate in biology with research into how trees flourish in the wild, Simard continued to gather scientific evidence to underpin her different understanding of forests based on collaboration. Her take, she was to discover, had a lot in common with the age-old stories and knowledge of indigenous peoples. Simard sought and found the answer below the surface. Trees and fungi form underground symbiotic associations known as *mycorrhizae*, networks of hyphae that extend for miles. The fungi even grow into the tree roots. In exchange for this connection, the fungi are given sugars that the trees create via photosynthesis and store in their green leaves. Among other phenomena, Simard examined the interactions between Douglas firs and paper birches. Her field research revealed that instead of competing, the two species in fact exchange carbon, nitrogen and sugars. The researcher has explained in interviews that she received little support from her mostly male colleagues, with the exception of her supervisor. And foresters would dismiss her interest in interaction at the expense of growth, yield and profit as very girlie. After decades of opposition, Simard's findings are now widely recognised and she is a professor in forest ecology at the University of British Columbia.

Simard's first publications in leading journals such as *Nature* date back several decades. In an article published in 1997, she effectively summed up what was then a rather alternative view of the functioning of forests: 'the theory that plant community dynamics operate mainly within the constraints of resource supply should be reformulated to consider mutualism between plants and their mycorrhizal fungi, as well as microbially mediated resource sharing.' Together with her research team, Simard found countless forms of cooperation in the forest. Old trees with deep roots extract water from the soil, which they then share with young, struggling trees. Hormones and alarm signals – to warn against predatory insects in the vicinity, for example – also flow from tree to tree via the mycorrhizal network. It makes sense then that she uses the term 'mother tree': the oldest trees in the forest look after new trees. And while direct descendants are given the most support, the others receive their fair share too – as if the mother tree knows that her progeny thrive in a complex union with other trees.

Simard's research challenges the paradigm of modern science, which rests on the worldview that took shape during the seventeenth century and focuses on individuals, conceived as separate atoms – whether these are the economically active, as in Adam Smith and his invisible hand (which posits that society is best off with selfish individuals who compete in a free market), or political philosopher Thomas Hobbes' men who are 'as wolves to other men'. Within this paradigm, most of the research by biologists since Darwin has been done from the perspective of a single species. The emphasis was on the survival of the fittest and later also on 'the selfish gene'. That focus, Simard writes, makes us blind: 'I'd been taught in the university to take apart the ecosystem, to reduce it into its parts, to study the trees and plants and soils in isolation, so that I could look at the forest objectively.' This working method would have made Simard a successful researcher, but it was not long before she realised that this framework made it 'almost impossible for a study of the diversity and connectivity of a whole ecosystem to get into print'.[61] Her stubbornness paid off. And we now have evidence that the wondrous underground symbiosis between plant roots, fungi and bacteria is a feature of just about every ecosystem on Earth.

The dominant, competition-based mindset has not only been shattered in forestry, but in quite a few other areas of society as well. Social interaction is one of them. Are we inherently competitive, or are we predisposed to work together? In the Dutch-speaking world, Dirk Van Duppen and Johan Hoebeke have brought together an impressive slew of studies in *De supersamenwerker* (The Super Collaborator). Their conclusion is persuasive: humans are social beings, collaborators, both generous and empathetic. Our social circumstances determine which qualities – be it collaboration or selfishness – prevail. These new insights debunk the persistent myth that human nature has evolved to be competitive and selfish. The book provides convincing evidence that collaboration and solidarity are key principles at work in the evolution of creatures in nature and humans in society.

It is therefore high time to base our thinking about human beings, the future of society and the relationship between humans and nature on a more realistic view of both mankind and the world. That includes a different perspective on our *way of being*. Of course, people can be racist and belligerent – newspaper headlines speak for themselves – but evolution has also made us social beings, hardwired to cooperate. This new understanding is informed by systems thinking, which helps us move beyond the reductionist approach. Philosopher Maria Puig de la Bellacasa captures it well when she writes that we need new ways of thinking 'to heal from the manic drive to dissect the togetherness that we perceive'.[62]

4. Another way of being: autonomy in connection

This brings us to the keywords associated with our new view of humanity: relationships, connectedness, empathy, solidarity and dependence. Suited and booted businessmen – to use a cliché – like to forget, but nobody grows up without having been cared for. All new-born babies are helpless and dependent on care and love. That is not a shortcoming, but the reality of human nature. As social beings, we grow up in a web of relationships; we become who we are through countless interactions. That is one of the pertinent points of feminist critique, put very well by the Swedish journalist Katrine Marçal: 'Without care *children* can't grow, the *sick* won't get healthy (…) and the old can't live. Being cared for by others is the medium through which *we learn cooperation, empathy, respect, self-discipline and thoughtfulness. These are fundamental life skills*.'[63]

Human beings want to care and be cared for. This allows us to work on a vision of the future that transcends the dominant view in our society, but without being naïve. We can only put caring at the heart of our lives if we restructure the world. Competition and competitiveness will never disappear. It is our environment that helps determine what kind of behaviour reigns supreme. So imagine designing society in such a way that competitiveness does not push care away, but that instead we start competing to offer the best possible care. This can make competition a force for good that enables us to take increasingly better care of one another and the planet.

Fortunately, the realisation that macho individualism – 'look, I don't need anyone' – is of no benefit to society is gaining ground. Dutch theatre maker Rebekka de Wit wrote a veritable *Declaration of Dependence* in 2019, in which she critiqued the prevailing notion that independence is the greatest good:

> 'It is strange: our social structures make us more dependent than ever and yet we are pretty successful at keeping this dependence out of the picture. (...) Why do we maintain a kind of illusion of independence for one another, day in day out? This illusion inevitably saddles us with existential problems, just as it seems to justify a great many political decisions, at every new climate conference.'[64]

Of course, that is not to say that autonomy – our emancipation into critical beings, capable of reflection and choices – is not a good thing. If so, de Wit would never have been able to write her essay. But the question is: how do we define this autonomy?

Interestingly, the early ecological theorists regarded autonomy as a collective practice, as the communal, joyful shaping of society. To redefine autonomy in this way, contemporary ecological thinkers draw on the concept of 'autonomy in connection'.[65] This ties in with the concept of freedom that de Wit refers to: the idea that our freedom lies in our highly personal desires, right here and now, is an illusion. What if you want to eat healthily, but you can only buy junk food in your neighbourhood? Or you would like to build a future for yourself in the country where you live, but you lack the appropriate documentation? Paradoxically, freedom is not something that is largely contingent on you as a person; it is more closely tied to whether society provides you with opportunities for personal development. It is the responsibility of the government and society to make it possible for you to develop the way you want to. At the very least that requires space to enter into a non-violent dialogue with others, so you can discover what you really want for yourself.

Autonomy in connection runs counter to the illusion of individuals who need nothing or nobody. Emancipation requires cooperation and often also bargaining for personal development opportunities. That was true for labourers in our corner of the world in the nineteenth century and still is for many oppressed groups across the globe. Autonomy in connection encompasses both a dimension of care and a need for social action. It also embraces the power of self-organisation: people taking their future into their own hands by establishing citizen collectives or commons. Think of those who want to push for renewable energy via cooperatives. While not necessarily pitting themselves against the government, they are certainly reacting to their leaders' failure to provide services fit for the future.

Commons are a beautiful manifestation of the recognition of our shared fate. We are connected with other life forms and dependent on one another, both to survive and to make a good life for ourselves. According to Jef Peeters, a researcher at KU Leuven, this teaches us, as social beings, how to act on the basis of a shared understanding of the world. Our cooperation creates feelings of mutual commitment and obligation.[66]

'Autonomy in connection' will of course always be defined in a particular context. In non-western societies, where individualisation is less extreme and kinship bonds are stronger, it will take other forms than it does here.

5. Regrounding ourselves

The French sociologist and philosopher Bruno Latour has highlighted just how obsolete our modern sense of self is. This self-image, in which humans view the world as a stage on which they play out their lives like actors, is underpinned by two preconceptions.

The first is that nature forms a passive background for human activity, a set that does not change unless the human dramaturg wants it to. If they do – and this is the second presumption – that backdrop will be readily changed, without it impacting the events on stage. Both assumptions are false. The growing number of ecological catastrophes make it clear that nature is not a passive set that humans can manipulate as they see fit. Nature has itself become an actor, which helps shape the theatrical play of humanity. It manifests itself daily in extreme temperatures or record precipitation.

Latour points out that the two dominant ways of coping with the reality of interconnectedness provide no answer. The first, the pursuit of the global – our constant sallying forth to conquer what lies beyond – is impossible on our finite Earth. As a result of economic globalisation, we now consume more than a single planet can give us. And when this way of life has claimed the entire Earth, there will be no safe haven anywhere. This means that the second frequent answer, localism, falling back on ourselves, offers no solution either: once the world has changed there is no turning back.

A new direction that *is* fit for the future and the polar opposite of the global-local axis involves regrounding ourselves, this time with an open mind about the world. By doing so the modern illusion of being independent of nature and being its master will transform into the earthly reality of mutual dependence. For Latour, mapping out the route that the ecological compass is inviting us to explore carries a powerful political message: 'To shift from one system to the other we shall have to learn to extricate ourselves from the reign of economization.'

This earthly dimension wants us to form a commitment to the land – to take care of it – while at the same time opening up to the world. And to do so in the crucial knowledge that humans are part of the complex living system that plays out on the Earth's crust and in the relatively thin layer around the Earth, the biosphere. This earthly perspective is different from the modern, as it no longer revolves around the planet in space – we are acutely aware of our precarious existence in this thin biosphere. Because that is what the illusion of modernity is: the belief that progress is possible by tearing down our set, that's to say, by damaging the biosphere. This 'stage set thinking' goes hand in hand with colonialism, which reduced both sections of the Earth and the people that lived there to a useable background, that claimed the lives of many and that continues to limit the development opportunities of many more to this day.

Rather than a farewell to modernity, this insight ought to help us shape a second modernity that openly acknowledges and learns from the mistakes of the first. At the same time, we cherish the good things brought to us by modern society rooted in the

Enlightenment: the importance of liberty, critical thought, the rule of law, education, science and technology, the rights of each individual.

6. A multitude of knowledge systems

Recalibrating our way of being in the world from a hierarchical top-down approach to an inclusive being-part-of-the-world will have consequences for our knowledge – that's to say, our ideas about the world that we consider to be true and just. As the example of Australia's colonisation shows, a dominant knowledge system has far-reaching implications. Modern western society attaches great importance to scientific knowledge accumulation. And with good reason: it has brought us a great deal. However, the problem is, firstly, that our society rejects all other forms of knowledge and knowledge systems, and, secondly, that it fixates on the reductionist model of scientific research. Western science reduces a system to its constituent parts, preferably in a lab, stripped of all context and possible interactions with other parts of the system.

Both critiques meet in Suzanne Simard's work: she encountered difficulties as she sought to pursue a holistic look at the land, and her findings resonate with the age-old knowledge of indigenous peoples. We have already seen that she struggled to get her systemic research published. It did not fit with the dissection of reality, so common in the dominant scientific domain. In *Finding the Mother Tree*, Simard cites Sm'hayetsk Teresa Ryan, a forest ecologist who studied with her. Ryan, of the Tsimshian, points out that recent research and the resulting new forestry practices reflect the insights and traditions of indigenous peoples. To them, it is clear that 'everything is interconnected', and that some of the cooperation occurs underground. The Menominee, who have been logging sustainably for 150 years, provide a concrete example. To them, sustainability means 'thinking in terms of whole systems, with all their interconnections, consequences and feedback loops'. This means, for instance, leaving the eldest trees – the grandmothers, as Simard would call them – in place without it reducing the forest's profitability.[67]

Acknowledging that, over the years, many indigenous peoples have built up an extensive body of ecological knowledge about living in synergy with biodiverse environments is of course not the same as idealising it. Being open to other perspectives and relationships with the world we are part of goes hand in hand with retaining our critical faculties.

7. The need for a new frame of reference

In his beautiful text 'De stilte in de storm' (The silence in the storm), eco-philosopher Jan Mertens points out that emotions such as sadness are more or less taboo in the climate debate.[68] His observation more generally reflects our performance-oriented culture, in which everybody is the *entrepreneur* of the self, the mood upbeat and success the only logical outcome. Yet today's ecological catastrophes evoke feelings of fear and sadness in many. When Greta Thunberg spoke at the World Economic Forum in Davos, she expressed the sentiments of quite a few young people:

> 'Adults keep saying we owe it to the young people to give them hope. But I don't want your hope, I don't want you to be hopeful. I want you to panic, I want you to feel the fear I feel every day. And then I want you to act, I want you to act as you would in a crisis. I want you to act as if the house was on fire, because it is.'[69]

Fear and sadness are perfectly normal emotions when your house is on fire. In fact, anything else would be weird. And, as Thunberg suggests, those emotions need not have a crippling effect. On the contrary. Mertens quotes the American writer, academic and environmental campaigner Joanna Macy: 'The pain you feel is born of your deep love for the world. It's an expression of our intrinsic connectedness with all life. In owning this pain and recasting it as compassion, we find a renewed strength that we can draw on to heal the world.'[70]

The Dutch broadcaster and humanist chaplain Evanne Nowak sums it up nicely by saying that the Anthropocene, as a distressing epoch of loss, calls for a new structure of feeling, a new way of experiencing things, which helps us recognise what is at stake:

> 'This age demands the courage to speak, to admit confusion and not-knowing and to face up to the extent of our problems. We ought to change conversational norms such as optimism, relativism and denial, slow down the debate and create an in-between space in which vulnerability is permitted and we get to address the questions that keep us and others awake at night.'[71]

Nowak explicitly recommends that we learn to mourn ecological breakdown, as those feelings have transformative qualities. At the same time, she reminds us to be aware of our position. Tears for climate loss can be 'white tears': the privileged western individual realising in shock that their bubble of prosperity is bursting. Suffering and injustice have been around for centuries, not least because of western imperialism. But the end of the illusion of western invulnerability can foster an openness in which climate despair is linked to the pain of age-old exploitation, racism and colonialism. Ecological mourning as a collective practice can help shape our identity and connect us to who and what we value. Nowak here draws on the ideas of American philosopher Judith Butler:

> 'What grief displays (...) is the thrall in which our relations with others hold us, in ways that we cannot always recount or explain (...), in ways that challenge the very notion of ourselves as autonomous and in control.'[72]

Inspired by Dutch sociologist Willem Schinkel, we want to argue for a politics of mourning. Being mindful of our inextricable connectedness is the antithesis of the capitalist pursuit of profit, which is based on the fiction that each one of us, individually, must shoulder our responsibility. Mourning may give us a different way of being in the world, a chance for humans to be social beings integrated with all other life forms. In fact, it is telling to see what we consider '*unmournable*'. Why don't we care to mark the loss of the ancient living environments of indigenous peoples? If the dominant western worldview regards the non-western and non-human other as *unmournable* – in a hard form of *othering* – it is high time we expose and transcend this cultural pattern of denial. The entire spectrum of hierarchies that Val Plumwood identified, the master narrative, attests to the fact that we have forgotten to think and feel that we are connected to all other life forms.

To Schinkel, this collective mourning is a challenge to the existing order, a challenge that is expressed, for example, in the Black Lives Matter protests. The grief for the many lives that have been lost has birthed a socio-critical movement that demands an end to racialised oppressive systems. All over the world, the BLM network seeks to redress the huge inequality of opportunity by stating, quite simply, that black lives matter too.

Intermezzo

For those familiar with Suzanne Simard's research and au fait with environmental philosophy, the life and work of Aldo Leopold may need little introduction. One of the founders of the conservation movement in the United States, he wrote in his seminal 1949 book *A Sand County Almanac* that instead of conquerors of the land-community, human beings ought to become members and citizens of it. We are connected with and dependent on other parts of the natural world.

While Simard started her career in a modern commercial logging business, Leopold started out as a forest ranger. One of his jobs was the extermination of predators to protect cattle and game. One day, he came across wolves in the forest:

> 'I was young then, and full of trigger-itch; *I thought that because fewer wolves meant more deer, that no wolves would mean hunters' paradise.*'

It cost at least one she-wolf her life. The 'fierce green fire dying in her eyes' would haunt Leopold for the rest of his days. He describes the incident in the essay 'Thinking Like a Mountain'. The title alone suggests that you can only understand the working of an ecosystem – such as a socio-ecological system of people living in a mountain valley – if you take account of its many intricate connections, interactions and dependencies. Once the wolves have disappeared from the forest, the forest itself may disappear. Without natural enemies, the deer will devour all the greenery.

Leopold sums up the crux of his *land ethics* in the preface to his book:

> 'That land is a community is the basic concept of ecology, but that land is to be loved and respected is an extension of ethics. That land yields a cultural harvest is a fact long known, but latterly often forgotten.'[73]

8. Caring as a collective mission

Who do we want to take care of? Acknowledging that we exist in-and-through relationships gives us an answer to that question. Acknowledging that we are at one with life forces us to look after the plurality of life forms and encourages active solidarity. It transcends what we traditionally define as 'care'. Think of parents raising their children, people – mostly women – doing the cooking and cleaning in the home (and being responsible for what, in the capitalist production perspective, is seen as the 'reproduction of life'). This invisible labour is what keeps the economy, so-called productive labour, running. But care is so much more: an accurate definition of care allows us to dispel a few spurious divisions, such as that between productive and reproductive labour.

The definition of care proposed by Joan Tronto and Berenice Fisher continues to inspire progressive thinkers more than thirty years on:

> 'On the most general level, we suggest that caring be viewed as a species activity that includes everything that we do to maintain, continue, and repair our 'world' so that we can live in it as well as possible. That world includes our body, our selves, and our environment, all of which we seek to interweave in a complex, life-sustaining *web*.'[74]

This description suggests that care encompasses a broad spectrum of activities ('everything that we do'), including that which is traditionally thought of as care (maintaining life or the home), the politics of care and care for a good life (living as well as possible). In keeping with the relational image of man, the emphasis here is on how everything in the web of life is interconnected and interdependent.

In other words, care is much more than a moral stance, more than what we do in the private sphere or as a paid care worker. Care comprises three fundamental dimensions: the concrete work of *everyday maintenance* – who is cooking for you tonight, or who is putting the child or the elderly parent to bed? – *affective engagement* and *ethico-political obligation*.[75]

There is nothing idealistic about care and caring; it can be joyful as well as demanding, incredibly absorbing but also exploitative. The latter is particularly true in an unequal world in which women and carers from marginalised groups still experience discrimination. Under a collective approach to care, we would share and divide caring responsibilities. At the same time, we would have to take a critical look at our extractive economy, which exploits both the natural world and people. If we want to champion a caring society, we will have to fight this injustice in our existing living conditions instead of tacitly accepting them. In that sense, an ethics of care is a collective responsibility, a response to the neoliberal belief in

'Smith's invisible hand' or the mantra 'work hard play hard'. One way of achieving this is by placing care at the heart of both the public debate and our everyday choices. We are not fully rational and self-determining selves, who take care decisions based on universal principles, independent of any physicality or kinship. Have you ever heard anyone say: 'inspired by philosopher John Rawls' theory of justice I'm going to take care of my neighbour and join an NGO for global solidarity'? What people do they do out of a sense of collectivity and engagement. As our discussion of mourning showed, people's actions are rooted in social motives that are never entirely visible or obvious. So-called reproductive labour must no longer be secondary to 'more important matters', such as politics or the production and selling of goods. There is no excuse, there is never a license for not wanting to care.

9. Caring for more-than-human worlds

If we subscribe to a relational image of the world – and accept that we are part of a greater whole – we cannot confine care to humans alone. The collapse of biodiversity shows this to be a dead end. Taking our inspiration from Maria Puig de la Bellacasa, we translate this insight into care for *more-than-human worlds*.[76] The concept fits in seamlessly with the new way of being, the new knowledge system and the new structure of feeling, and it conveys the idea that our frame of reference remains, but is not limited to, the human aspect. It shows that we cannot differentiate between human and non-human care relationships. Those who care for the natural world care for humans. This is reflected in the objectives of the One Health approach. The planet and human beings are inextricably linked, as the Covid crisis has once again shown. This new position asks us to painstakingly *decentre* ourselves – to not always see humans as the centre of everything – yet remain very close to people in their particular and sometimes precarious circumstances. Decentring ourselves as humans and seeing ourselves first and foremost as embedded in the web of life with lots of different life forms does not relieve us of our accountability. On the contrary, the new way of being and the new insights force us to finally handle the complexity more responsibly. It is a complexity that keeps surprising us, that stuns us – as it did in Simard's story. Once you realise how intricate a forest is, you treat it more carefully and you want everybody else to do the same.

The description 'more-than-human worlds' also allows us to move beyond classic binary thinking, which in environmental philosophy focuses on questions such as: 'What is nature and what is culture? Is intrinsic value limited to humans or does it extend to the natural world? Can we still speak of nature in the Anthropocene?' The answer that transcends these dichotomies is clear. Even if everything on Earth has been touched by human activity, there is no need to declare nature dead. It may be more accurate to say that we live in *nature cultures*. Socio-ecological systems is another way to describe it. Of course nature still exists, but as the French anthropologist Philippe Descola stresses: 'Even the mighty Amazon Rainforest was shaped by thousands of years' worth of interventions by indigenous communities.' The nature-culture divide is far less clear-cut than we think, especially when we consider that humans have controlled fire for hundreds of thousands of years.[77] If we are to rise above this binary thinking, it makes more sense to speak of nature and culture as the two extremes of a continuum. All communities offer their own interpretation of the two concepts and the way they relate to one another.

We are dealing with an ontological shift – a shift in our concept of being – based on interconnectedness. We no longer view the non-human as purely an object (the mountain and the wolf in Leopold, the tree and the fungus in Simard) and humans as the sole subject. This has nothing to do with romanticising the natural world, or on the contrary, wanting to completely manipulate it. What does this mean for the careful handling of more-than-human worlds? Puig de la Bellacasa finds inspiration in three interlocking principles from permaculture: *earth care*, *people care* and *fair share*. The application of these three will always call for a situated response – each context is different – and a collective dialogue. 'Who do we want to take care of?' is never a question that just floats in the ether; it is always embedded in very concrete situations. Answering the question from this perspective also means broadening the definition of care: it is not about what *we* do just so *we* can live our best possible lives on Earth. Our world encompasses the specific nature culture, the interconnectedness that ensures the conservation of the biosphere and the preservation and renewal of life. The more we recognise our dependence on one another, the more acutely we acknowledge the need for care in more-than-human relationships.

10. A caring democracy that drives the economy

To Joan Tronto it is obvious: if we want to create a caring society, we need a caring democracy. Care requires time and resources and these are very unequally distributed in the world. Setting about creating a caring democracy, with an emphasis on citizenship and values such as equality and justice, means actively resisting relationships of extraction, exploitation and oppression. A caring democracy that is based on a participatory model will engage in a dialogue about the allocation of care responsibilities. The key question is how the principles of democracy can be brought to bear on the reality of various dependency relationships, and how the various hierarchies in our society can be eradicated in the distribution of care responsibilities.[78]

This politicised take on care allows us to avoid the pitfall of essentialism: just because it is still mainly women who shoulder care responsibilities – due to unequal power relations – does not mean that caring essentially 'belongs' to women. That would depoliticise the concept of 'care', keep it in the private sphere, leave the role of men out of the equation… which would maintain the status quo, serving vested interests. That said, rejecting this essentialism does not mean denying the present-day and historical role of women in relation to care. On the contrary. This position allows us to deploy care in a politicising and strategic way. We can do so, as Tronto explains, by viewing care as a political concept, which assumes that all roles in society – whether of men or women – are open to change and up for democratic debate. For Tronto, care is central to any definition of a good society. Care can therefore not be restricted to the private sphere or to women alone. This then moves the question of how we can distribute the work and responsibility of care on the basis of justice and equality to the heart of the democratic debate.

A central issue in the discussion about a caring society and the caring democracy that goes with it – perhaps even the fundamental question – is the relationship between democracy and the economy. It is of course fine to try and strengthen care within the current economic system. For some people it may make a world of difference in the short term. But this may well be a case of symptom relief. As the sociologist Saskia Sassen documents in her book *Expulsions*, predatory capitalism and its global capital flows inevitably exclude people, land and nature from society. A large percentage of the value created by many goes to a small group of wealthy people who live off interest, share prices and speculation. Neoliberal capitalism rests on the plunder of the natural world and the exploitation of labour in the Global South, while in the rest of the world the number of precarious jobs and zero-hours contracts is going up. All this is connected: because of the import of cheap consumer goods – made possible, in part, by child labour in Bangladesh – there is no need for our wages in the west to go up. The outcome? The added value from the increase in productivity tends to end up in the hands of those who hold capital, while the wage labourers have to make do with the crumbs. It leaves the emancipation of women via the labour market with a bad aftertaste, seeing as it takes place in the context of a crumbling welfare state in which the importance of purchasing power to obtain care keeps growing. The restoration of the twentieth-century welfare state is not a forward-looking option either: the painful truth is that social security is funded through an economic model that undermines the foundations of a liveable Earth, while for centuries it has also been extracting value from other communities and living environments in the Global South. The key mission of a truly caring society is becoming abundantly clear: we need to set about creating a different economic model.

Neoliberal capitalism is not an economic subsystem of society that conforms to democratic decisions. With principles such as commodification having already permeated every facet of our lives, it is more likely to try and manipulate democracy to serve its own interests. The stability of western nation states with huge government debt partly depends on the credit ratings that private companies assign to the financial markets. Capitalism, as the inspiring American sociologist Nancy Fraser explains, is not simply a part of our society. Capitalism structures society and tries to impose an institutional social order based on divisions such as those between so-called productive and reproductive (or domestic) labour and between society and non-human nature. So heeding the analysis of ecofeminists and adopting Tronto's definition of care, we must conclude that only a complete overhaul of the economy into a caring economy can bring about our evolution into a caring society.

The foundations of the economy (and economics as an academic discipline) must be radically altered if we are to realise this transformation. As many ecofeminists and ecological economists have highlighted, the point of the economy is not to satisfy the fickle desires of consumers (provided they have the required spending power), but to meet *the human need to pursue a good life* within the limits of what the planet can support while safeguarding the opportunities of future generations. This returns us to the original meaning of economy, Aristotle's *oikonomia*: the art of household management, of maintaining one's house, the entire living planet Earth. From this perspective, speculation on the future price of food, for example, is not a rational investment, but an immoral practice that ought to be democratically banned.

This brings us to a second central issue: democracy must wrest back control of the economy. Again, this has nothing to do with an economy planned from the top-down, but everything to do with the democratic adoption of rules to protect the public interest. In that respect, it is downright disgraceful that the financial sector, having triggered the biggest economic crisis since World War II in 2008, has still not come under the control of democratic bodies. The separation of retail and investment banking, a fundamental measure in response to the Great Depression in the 1930s, has not yet been reintroduced. The economy (including the world of finance) must absolutely be democratically embedded. Unfair trade agreements continue to consolidate the subordinate role of very low-income countries in the Global South, which, to make matters worse, are also burdened by enormous debt. Much of that debt needs to be written off if we are to have equal opportunities for all countries on Earth.

The key question raised by this second central issue is which of the three basic forms of social organisation we prioritise. The neoliberal order is characterised by the belief that the *market* is the most efficient form of organisation, scepticism about the government and its public services and disdain for citizens' self-organisation in commons. However, the Covid crisis has shown that giving the market free rein puts society and the natural world at risk. It is entirely possible for the *government* to regulate the economy, just like *citizens* can organise themselves quickly and efficiently – just think of local and urban support networks. We must learn the necessary lessons from this and explicitly ask ourselves which forms of commodification we allow in which social domains. There is nothing wrong with markets per se – they have been around since time immemorial without dominating the entire social order – except that we have evolved from a society with markets to a market society, as the social philosopher Karl Polanyi aptly put it.[79] This is why most people think it makes perfect sense for listed companies to buy up residential care homes with the aim of getting a return on their investment year on year. This profit-driven objective is at odds with investing as much as possible in care staff. The same reasoning applies to education.

This presents us with the fundamental challenge of *re-embedding* the economy in a democratic way. Rather than a purely theoretical issue, it is a pressing daily concern in many areas. The political and social conflict surrounding the housing market in Berlin is a good example of this battle for the democratic re-embedding of the economy. Applied to housing, the game of supply and demand within the dominant economic system ensures that all consumers have access to a suitable and affordable home. Reality shows this to be false. International hedge funds, project developers and platform companies such as Airbnb regard houses as investments – they might as well be washing powder. If it is more profitable to keep homes empty, to charge exorbitant prices or to make them exclusively available to tourists, these companies will effectively do that. And every year the growing housing shortage is affecting more people. To counter this, Berlin's Green city council decided to freeze the rents of existing homes for five years. But because this clashed with the way things are normally done, a judge ruled that only the federal government had the authority to do so. Meanwhile, during a second phase, enough signatures have been collected to force a referendum aimed at expropriating big real estate companies.[80] While set to be a tough fight, it clearly demonstrates that the struggle to curb commodification is alive and well. And as more and more residents in other cities – in Amsterdam, for example, where the council has also initiated action against Airbnb – likewise refuse to put up with the colonisation of homes by market players, the chance grows of an interurban coalition with more clout and impact.

11. An economy that looks after people's real needs

It is fascinating to see that the topic of living well within planetary boundaries is receiving more and more attention in the academic community. The research also shows that it is an illusion to think that an economy addicted to growth, based on competition and therefore inequality, will ever achieve this target. Recent studies into 'the good life' have rediscovered, among other work, the model of the Chilean economist Manfred Max-Neef. He developed it as a scholar in Chile in the 1980s and 1990s to allow grassroots communities in Latin America to take their future into their own hands and to break away from failing neoliberal top-down formulas. His *human scale development* approach, the fruit of research carried out by a transdisciplinary team in several Latin American nations, is now used the world over. Crucial to this theoretical framework is the difference between the needs themselves and how they are met by so-called *satisfiers*. The latter can be political structures as well as social practices and forms of organisation. The large-scale study shows that there are, in essence, nine fundamental human needs: subsistence (health, food, shelter, clothing), protection (care, solidarity, work), affection (self-esteem, love, care, solidarity), understanding (studying, learning, analysing), participation (accepting responsibilities, having rights and duties), idleness (playing, relaxing, having fun), creation (imagination, work, curiosity), identity (the sense of belonging, differentiation, self-esteem) and freedom (autonomy, self-determination, equality). Whereas the basic needs are universal, the choice of satisfiers is culturally defined. This kind of holistic approach illustrates that there are alternatives to the dominant, market-based fulfilment of needs.[81]

It is interesting to see how Max-Neef's principles chime with the main tenets of ecofeminism:

1. The economy is not about material things or GNP, but about people and their opportunities for adequately satisfying their fundamental needs. And unless we adopt other criteria for economic success, criteria based on well-being, we will never get there.
2. The economy is about people's vital needs, basic requirements that are limited in number and finite, and therefore not about insatiable consumer wants. Until we see care and domestic labour as building blocks of every economic system, we will keep going round in circles.

3. The economy can be understood through systems thinking, which stresses that people are relational beings who live in permanent mutual interaction with their more-than-human worlds. This concept starts not from the almighty consumer, but from the fundamental interdependence between people and the web of life they are part of.

The crucial question here remains: how do we put this into practice in today's complex society? The likes of Jason Hickel, Giorgos Kallis, Kate Raworth and Julia Steinberger have been developing highly relevant ideas in recent years. The essential conceptual shift, one with huge practical potential, is the turn away from the focus on satisfying fickle consumer wants within an economy addicted to growth to meeting human needs through so-called *provisioning systems* within the limits of our planet. This shift ties in seamlessly with contemporary ecofeminist theories:

> 'To define economics *as the study* of social provisioning is to emphasize that at its root, economic activity involves the ways people organize themselves collectively to get a living. (…) *Social provisioning need not* be done through the *market*; it need not be done for selfish or self-interested reasons, although neither of these is inconsistent with social provisioning, either.'[82]

How does this play out on a concrete level? A large-scale research project called Living Well Within Limits, led by Professor Julia Steinberger, examines which socio-ecological forms of provisioning would allow all people on Earth to create a decent life for themselves within the limits of the planet.[83] The comprehensive statistical analysis of a big data set is yielding some unambiguous conclusions: some provisioning factors almost always have a positive impact, while others are consistently harmful in a range of circumstances. The provisions that were found to be favourable include: public service quality, democracy, income equality, access to electricity and healthcare. Conversely, extractivism and economic growth are identified as detrimental. A plant-based diet, a move towards smarter construction and thorough insulation of buildings and the transition from individual to collective and sustainable transport are important and concrete changes in the provisioning systems that are already being implemented. Think of the trend in many cities of banning cars in favour of public transport, bikes and pedestrians.

These findings are in tune with the work of economic anthropologist Jason Hickel, which shows that once a particular, not very high level of income has been achieved a good quality of life depends first and foremost on good healthcare and education, as well as low levels of inequality. This means that, in defiance of the dominant discourse, abandoning the pursuit of economic growth, beyond a certain level of welfare, is ecologically imperative and socially desirable.

In his book *Less Is More*, Hickel specifically addresses the assumption, made by quite a few economists and policy makers, that a rise in GDP is crucial to our welfare. Hickel shows that the relationship between growth and human progress is not as straightforward as is generally assumed. Beyond a certain point, a higher GDP will not necessarily improve our well-being. The same is true for the historical development of western nations. For many years it was thought that the increase in average life expectancy, such as that in the United Kingdom from the nineteenth century onwards, was mainly due to the rise in GDP and average income. In order to guarantee this in the future, the economy had to keep growing. Recent research casts serious doubt on this equation of growth with progress. Historians now agree that people's life expectancy increased drastically not because of economic growth in itself, but thanks to clean drinking water and better sanitation. The role of social movements in this should not be underestimated either:

> 'These movements delivered not only public sanitation systems but also, in the years that followed, public healthcare, vaccination coverage, public education, public housing, better wages and safer working conditions. According to research by the historian Simon Szreter,

> access to these public goods [...] had a significant positive impact on human health, and spurred soaring life expectancy through the twentieth century.'[84]

The same phenomenon occurred in the United States. Following water sanitation measures between 1900 and 1936, child mortality dropped by 75 per cent, and overall mortality rates by 50 per cent.[85] After improved sanitation, access to healthcare is the prime catalyst for higher life expectancy. Education plays a key role, too. This means that in countries where universal public goods are not yet in place, economic growth is needed to provide these basic provisions. But beyond a certain level, growth will not necessarily boost welfare:

> 'Over and over again, the empirical evidence shows that it is possible to achieve high levels of human development without high levels of GDP.'[86]

Hickel's ideas have a lot in common with those of Max-Neef: public wellbeing can be realised in ways other than through endless economic growth. Once basic services are met, there is room to focus on cooperation, coexistence and community spirit. Hickel cites a study by Stanford University School of Medicine that shows that, besides the aforementioned provisions, people who are embedded in robust networks (of family, friends and neighbours) tend to live longer.[87]

These research findings enable us to sketch the outlines of a political programme that targets the transformation to a caring society and a caring economy. Ample, high-quality public services are crucial building blocks, as are a high degree of income equality and low levels of extractivism. An economy that breaks with exploitation and extraction will have to focus on those basic, and finite, needs. Nobody needs three homes to meet their housing needs, and besides, living in a space-efficient and socially rich co-housing project may well give the most satisfaction.

This means choosing an economic system based on sufficiency. It is the positive answer to the soulless 'ever more, ever faster', a response that stands for quality of work and life and the right to self-determination. It ties in with the well-known Brundtland definition of sustainability. While the first part, '*development that meets the needs of the present*,' has become a hollow phrase, it is the second clause that really gets to the heart of the matter: '*without compromising the ability of future generations to meet their own needs*.' It sets out two basic requirements: priority must be given to the needs of the world's poor, and we must recognise that the current state of technology and social organisation means limits on the (over)use of the natural world. When we acknowledge those limits – and climate breakdown is a potent daily reminder – we have no choice but to embrace the sufficiency economy.

12. Decolonising the economy

This future-oriented blueprint of the economy ties in seamlessly with the need to decolonise the economic system. One community's needs must never be met at the expense of another. Those that take from a certain place – as an extractive economy does – also remove life chances from that locale. As philosopher Achille Mbembe puts it, 'for centuries we conflated civilisation with industrial civilisation,' which inevitably meant that other-than-industrial civilisations were deemed to be of lesser value.[88] According to Plumwood, this is yet another example of *othering*: everything or everyone different from the norm is seen as inferior. Mbembe points to the relationship between slavery on plantations, colonial over-exploitation and current forms of land and resource grabbing. Land grabbing rests on the same principle that underpinned the British colonisation of Australia: the failure to recognise other systems of use and ownership, however ancient they are. The economic system of the plantation and today's extractivism share the same basic structure: 'The denial that humans and the environment are connected and that all forms of life have the right to exist.'[89] Alma De Walsche stresses that, for Mbembe, the key concepts are care and recovery now that so much has been destroyed. Decolonisation calls for an entirely different logic and a new set of relations between human and non-human beings at a moment when life itself is under threat. And, tied to the ethics of care, efforts at *reparative justice*. Reality shows that work in this area has yet to begin. Reparations for the abuse of enslavement have never been made – unlike the reverse, in Haiti. While France has never compensated Haiti for the damage it inflicted as coloniser and slave trader, in 1825 the European nation – in exchange for recognising the island's independence – demanded a substantial sum from the Haitian government to recompense the French state and its colonists for their losses during the Haitian Revolution. Having little choice at the time, Haiti accepted the terms. However, the country could only pay by borrowing from French and American banks. This meant that in 1915, for example, more than a century after independence, 80 per cent of Haiti's budget went to repaying these banks. The payments continued until 1947, at which stage the country was virtually bankrupt. Ironically, this makes the first independent black nation the only one to date to have paid 'reparations' for slavery (in the opposite direction).[90] Some movements are now demanding that France repay this money.

Decolonising means subscribing to the ecological view that creates new relationships between human and non-human beings as well as new economic systems that undo othering and thus transcend differences based on race, gender or nation state. Mbembe, echoing the insights offered by ecofeminism, argues that 'we have to break the vicious circles of the dichotomies and fashion new identities from the multitude of archives that have been passed down to us.' As Alma De Walsche puts it, for Mbembe this means going in search of new ways of thinking and new, empathy-based relationships with all life forms. 'There is ... *no world* except by way of naming, delegation, *mutuality*, and *reciprocity*,' he writes in the epilogue to *Critique of Black Reason*. This involves working on trans-local solidarity, and facilitating, instead of obstructing, the conditions that allow people everywhere to bring about their emancipation.

An economics based on sufficiency, starts from a 'fair Earth share for everyone', that is to say an equal distribution of access to and use of resources within the limits of the planet, as well as a fair distribution of greenhouse gas emissions. This requires both the discontinuation of fossil fuel use and the dematerialisation of the economy by a factor of ten. It chimes with what Kate Raworth describes as the 'safe operating space for humanity': a domain that is free and just for all, in which social rights are guaranteed while we remain within the limits of natural, life-sustaining systems. A sufficiency economy is in effect the school of efficiency's necessary twin. It is obviously good that domestic appliances have the best possible energy ratings, but if we convert the energy savings to cheap flights, we are doomed. These so-called rebound effects negate a substantial portion of the efficiency gains,[91] and only the specification of 'ecological ceilings', the quantity of raw materials an economy can use, can counter them.

Ecological justice, for both current and future generations, requires rich households to consume less so they free up the necessary environmental space for poorer demographics to meet their needs. A single figure illustrates both the challenge and the urgency: worldwide the richest 10 per cent are responsible for roughly half of all consumer-related greenhouse gas emissions, while the poorest 50 per cent account for only 10 per cent of emissions.

Kate Raworth has said in recent lectures: 'Every country – whether rich or poor – is a "developing country".' There are some high-income countries where the average life is good, but where the pressure on the environment and the extraction levels are unsustainable. Then there are countries categorised as low-income that have difficulties providing the best living conditions, but that have very little impact on the planet's natural resources. Each country then has a very specific development trajectory, influenced by its historical and geographical positioning, whether it is one of the richest or poorest. The historical fact of 'ecological debt' must be factored into this: the wealth of industrialised nations in the North is rooted in the plunder of natural resources in the South and the excessive use of the environmental space, for instance through greenhouse gas emissions. It is yet another argument in favour of decolonising the economic system as fast and fully as possible, which should include the agreement of forms of reparation.

Such an economy is conceivable only from a post-capitalist, post-growth perspective. Rather than putting our energy into precisely labelling this future economic system, it would be more productive to use systems thinking to describe the project, define its potential building blocks and – even more importantly – test it. It is up to high-income countries to continue to ensure a good standard of living despite a drastic reduction in the energy and material required by the economy. The cornerstones of such an economy include a shorter working week, shared goods and services (such as bicycle and car sharing), durable and reparable appliances, affordable public services (so purchasing power plays no role in public transport, healthcare or education), fair taxation, etc.

Systems thinking shows clearly that a new policy in just one area will make little difference. System change is possible only with drastic measures across a range of spheres – measures that reinforce and amplify one another. Think of production and consumption patterns, the legislative framework, taxation and the strengthening of democratic participation.

Systems thinking draws on intersectional thought to reveal that forms of exclusion and exploitation go hand in hand and tend to affect specific groups more than others. People on low incomes have fewer opportunities on the housing and labour markets, with women of colour on a low income particularly hard hit. And the list goes on. We could start by aiming for clusters of measures that convert intersections into synergies, working to create nodes of empowerment. To illustrate this: free childcare provision during school holidays by and for local parents, in buildings and premises made available by a school or local government is a fine example of a commons that can make a world of difference; on a global level, a wealth and speculation tax can reduce inequality and generate funds to give low-income countries maximum support in their efforts to tackle the drastic consequences of climate change.

However, an ethics of care does not just encompass the actions of groups of people or of society as a whole. In practical terms, it can also be translated into a duty of care for businesses. Existing international guidelines already stipulate that companies must do everything in their power to prevent human rights violations and environmental pollution. But because these guidelines are not enforceable, they amount to a dead letter. The alternative would be to include the duty of care for businesses in binding legislation. The European Commission made a start in 2020, when it announced plans to introduce mandatory due diligence laws for business supply chains. As we know, the rare earth metals in our smartphones are linked to child labour and ecological destruction in the Global South. Meanwhile, courts in several countries have sentenced governments in so-called climate cases, with judges ordering them to come up with more ambitious climate policies because they have a duty of care towards the country's residents, and in particular the children.

13. A worldwide coalition for a new eco-social contract

A politics of care aimed at transformation can only succeed within an overarching political framework. We will have to look at how we can replace the social contract of the twentieth-century welfare state – which evidently failed to shoulder care for the entire world – with a new eco-social contract for more-than-human worlds. The UNRISD (United Nations Research Institute for Social Development) has drawn up a concrete proposal for this, which considers the planet's boundaries as well as human rights in a broader spectrum.[92] Its focus is on intersectional policy to reach groups that are currently facing various disadvantages. The new eco-social contract addresses seven themes, and is fundamentally different from its twentieth-century counterpart on the following points:

1. *Human rights for all*, including those that are frequently marginalised.
2. *A progressive fiscal contract*, which raises sufficient funding for climate action and distributes the financial burdens fairly.
3. *Transforming economies and societies*, in the realisation that this is crucial to halting climate breakdown and fostering social inclusion and equality.
4. *A contract with nature*, informed by our recognition that as human beings we are part of a global ecosystem. This also involves the protection of ecological processes and biodiversity.
5. *Decolonising*, taking inspiration from the capabilities, social values and indigenous knowledge in the Global South, while also eradicating historical injustices.
6. *Gender justice*, stressing the equality of men and women, sharing production and reproduction activities equally between all genders and granting equal respect and rights to all sexual orientations and gender identities.
7. *New forms of solidarity*, on the strength of bottom-up approaches to change, which bring together social movements and progressive alliances of scientists, policy makers and activists.

Within the care perspective that we set out with the help of systems thinking in this essay, decolonisation involves much more than just the eradication of historical injustices. The goal of transitional justice requires changing the structures underlying the injustices and introducing mechanisms that facilitate a non-violent approach to conflict.

The successful adoption of such an eco-social contract depends on a worldwide coalition of the various movements and organisations that fight for freedom and emancipation. Their goals tie in perfectly with the care perspective, in which care 'includes everything that we do to maintain, continue, and repair our "world" so that we can live in it as well as possible'. It would be a motivating thought experiment to consider what unions, environmental and climate activists, women's movements and organisations such as Black Lives Matter might be able to do if they joined forces to form the liberation movement of the twenty-first century. Rather than 'strength through unity', it would unlock the power of diversity. We are fortunate that we get to stand on the shoulders of many eco-feminist thinkers, including Val Plumwood, who encapsulated the mission in the first few lines of what remains an inspiring classic:

> 'It is usually at the edges where the great tectonic plates of theory meet and shift that we find the most dramatic developments and

> upheavals. When four tectonic plates of liberation theory – those concerned with the oppressions of gender, race, class and nature – finally come together, the resulting tremors could shake the conceptual structures of oppression to their foundations.'

More than thirty years on from this powerful analysis, it is time to bring the tectonic plates in society together. Our future has not yet been determined – we can still take matters into our own hands. Our actions today and from this point forward will forge the path ahead. This essay aimed to centre radical care through the lens of intersectional ecofeminism in the hope that it would offer the necessary inspiration for realising that future in which care is not just something that is talked about, but also widely practised.

Bibliography

Arendt, H. (1958). *The Human Condition*. Chicago: University of Chicago Press.

Arikoglu, F., Scheepers, S., Koranteng Kumi, A. (2014). *Intersectioneel Denken: Handleiding voor professionelen die intersectionaliteit of kruispunt-denken in de eigen organisatie willen toepassen* (Intersectional thought: A manual for applying intersectionality to professional organisations). Brussels: Ella vzw.

Burgers, L., Meijer E., Nowak E. (2020). *De stem van de Noordzee. Een pleidooi voor vloeibaar denken* (The Voice of the North Sea: In praise of fluidity). Boom uitgevers, Amsterdam.

Crenshaw, K. (1989). 'Demarginalizing the Intersection of Race and Sex: A Black Feminist Critique of Antidiscrimination Doctrine, Feminist Theory and Antiracist Politics.' *University of Chicago Legal Forum*. 1, 139-167.

Crenshaw, K., interviewed in M.C. McCauley (27 September 2016). 'Intersectionality concerns transcend straight, white feminism.' *Baltimore Sun*. https://www.baltimoresun.com/features/women-to-watch/bal-intersectionality-baltimore-feminism-20160926-story

Descola P. (2021). *Une écologie des relations* (An ecology of relationships). Paris: CNRS Editions/De Vive Voix.

De Walsche A. (2021). 'Dekoloniseren: breken met het verleden of verbinden met de toekomst?' (Decolonising: breaking with the past, or linking up with the future?), *Oikos* 99, 3, 65-74.

de Wit, R. (2019). *Afhankelijkheidsverklaring* (Declaration of Dependence). Amsterdam: Atlas Contact.

European Environmental Bureau (EEB) and Women Engage for a Common Future (WECF) (2021). Why the European Green Deal needs ecofeminism. Moving from gender-blind to gender-transformative environmental policies. Heidegger, P., N. Lharaig, K. Wiese, A. Stock and R. Heffernan (eds.).

Fisher, B. & Tronto, J. (1990) 'Toward a Feminist Theory of Caring', in *Circles of Care*, Abel E. & Nelson, M. (eds.), 36-54. Albany, NY: SUNY Press.

Ghosh, A. (2016). *The Great Derangement. Climate Change and the Unthinkable.* Chicago: The University of Chicago Press.

Hache, E. (2016). *Reclaim. Receuil de Textes Écoféministes* (Reclaim. Anthology of ecofeminist texts). Paris: Éditions Cambourakis.

Harris, M. (2016). 'Ecowomanism. An Introduction.' *Worldviews: Global Religions, Culture, and Ecology*, 20(1), 5-14.

Hickel, J. (2021). *Less Is More. How Degrowth Will Save the World.* London: Heinemann.

Holemans, D. (2016). *Vrijheid & Zekerheid: Naar een sociaalecologische samenleving* (Freedom & Security: Towards a socio-ecological society). Berchem: EPO.

Holemans, D. (ed.) (2020). *Het Ecologisch Kompas* (The ecological compass). Berchem: EPO.

Holemans, D. (2021). 'Commons as Polanyian countermovement in neoliberal market society. A case study in Belgium', in *Community Development Journal.* https://academic.oup.com/cdj/advance-article-abstract/doi/10.1093/cdj/bsab007/6243392

hooks, b. (1989). *Talking Back: Thinking Feminist, Thinking Black*. London: Sheba.

Hunnicutt, G. (21 April 2020). 'Dr. Gwen Hunnicutt: Ecofeminism and the Ethics of Care.' *UNCG News*. https://news. uncg.edu/dr-gwen-hunnicutt-ecofeminism/

Intergovernmental Science-Policy Platform on Biodiversity and Ecosystem Services (IPBES) (2019). *Global assessment report on biodiversity and ecosystem services*. E.S. Brondizio, J. Settele, S. Díaz, and H.T. Ngo (eds). Bonn: IPBES secretariat.

Intergovernmental Panel on Climate Change (IPCC) (2021). *Climate Change 2021: The Physical Science Basis. Contribution of Working Group I to the Sixth Assessment Report of the Intergovernmental Panel on Climate Change*. Masson-Delmotte, V., P. Zhai, A. Pirani, S.L. Connors, C. Péan, S. Berger, N. Caud, Y. Chen, L. Goldfarb, M.I. Gomis, M. Huang, K. Leitzell, E. Lonnoy, J.B.R. Matthews, T.K. Maycock, T. Waterfield, O. Yelekçi, R. Yu and B. Zhou (eds.). Cambridge: Cambridge University Press.

Latour, B. (2018). *Down To Earth. Politics in the New Climatic Regime*. Cambridge: Polity.

Leopold, A. (1949). *A Sound County Almanac*. New York: Ballantine.

MacGregor, S. (2004). 'From Care to Citizenship: Calling Ecofeminism Back to Politics.' *Ethics & The Environment*. 9(1), 56-84.

Max-Neef, M. (1991). *Human Scale Development Conception, Application and Further Reflections*, New York/London: The Apex Press.

Marçal, K. (2015). *Who Cooked Adam Smith's Dinner? A Story About Women and Economics*. London: Portobello Books.

Meadows, D. (1999). 'Leverage Points: Places to Intervene in a System.' *The Sustainability Institute*, 1-19.

Mbembe, A. (2017). *Critique of Black Reason*. Durham, NC: Duke University Press.

Merchant, C. (1980). *The Death of Nature: Women, Ecology and the Scientific Revolution*. San Francisco: Harper & Row.

Mies, M. & Shiva, V. (2014). *Ecofeminism*. London and New York: Zed Books.

Misiedjan, D. (August 2021). 'Onderzoeker Daphina Misiedjan: klimaatproblemen zijn ongelijk verdeeld' (Researcher Daphina Misiedjan: climate problems affect us unequally). *Brainwash*. https://

www.brainwash.nl/bijdrage/klimaatproblemen-zijn-ongelijk-verdeeld

Muthuki, J. (2006). 'Challenging Patriarchal Structures: Wangari Maathai and the Green Belt Movement in Kenya.' *Agenda*, 20(69), 83-91.

Peeters, J. (2021). 'Economie in meervoud. Deel VII. Naar zorg als kern van de economie' (Economics multiplied. Part VII. Care at the heart of the economy). *Oikos* 98, 91-105.

Phillips, M. (2019). '"Daring to Care": Challenging Corporate Environmentalism.' *Journal of Business Ethics*, 156, 1151-1164.

Plumwood, V. (1993). *Feminism and the Mastery of Nature*. London: Routledge.

Power, M. (2004). 'Social provisioning as a starting point for feminist economics.' *Feminist Economics*, 10 (3), 3-19.

Puig de la Bellacasa, M. (2017). *Matters of Care. Speculative Ethics in More Than Human Worlds*. Minneapolis: University of Minnesota Press.

Purtschert, P. (June 2020). 'What can we learn from ecofeminists?' *Gender Campus*. https://www.gendercampus.ch/en/ blog/post/what-can-we-learn-from-ecofeminists

Rico, A. (2017). 'Gendered Ecologies and Black Feminist Futures in Wanuri Kahiu's *Pumzi*, Wangechi Mutu's *The End of Eating Everything* and Ibi Zoboi's *The Farming of Gods*.' *Wagadu: A Journal of Transnational Women's and Gender Studies*, 18, 81-99.

Roy, A. (3 April 2020). 'Arundhati Roy: The Pandemic is a Portal.' *Financial Times*. https://www.ft.com/content/10d8f5e8-74eb-11ea-95fe-fcd274e920ca

Sassen, S. (2014). *Expulsions*. Cambridge: Harvard University Press.

Schinkel, W. (2021). *Pandemocratie* (Pandemocracy). Amsterdam: Leesmagazijn.

Shiva, V. (1988). *Staying Alive: Women, Ecology and Survival in India*. New Delhi: Kali For Women.

Shiva, V. (1993). *Monocultures of the Mind: Perspectives on Biodiversity and Biotechnology*. London: Palgrave Macmillan.

Shiva, V. (2005). *Earth Democracy: Justice, Sustainability, and Peace*. Boston: South End Press.

Shiva, V. & Bandyopadhyay, J. (1986). 'The Evolution, Structure and Impact of the Chipko

Movement.' *Mountain Research and Development*, 6(2), 133-142.

Simard, S. (2021). *Finding the Mother Tree: Uncovering the Wisdom and Intelligence of the Forest.* London: Allen Lane.

Sturgeon, N. (1997). *The Nature Of Race. Indigenous Women And White Goddesses.* London and New York: Routledge.

Tronto, J. (1993). *Moral Boundaries: A Political Argument for an Ethic of Care.* New York: Routledge.

Tronto, J. (2017). 'There is an alternative: homines curans and the limits of neoliberalism' in *International Journal of Care and Caring* 1.1, 27-43.

Tutu, D. (3 April 2013). 'Who we are: Human uniqueness and the African spirit of Ubuntu.' Desmond Tutu, Templeton Prize 2013. https://youtu.be/owZtfqZ271w

Vogel, J., Steinberger, J.K., O'Neill, D.W., Lamb, W.F. & Krishnakumar, J. (2021). 'Socio-economic conditions for satisfying human needs at low energy use: an international analysis of social provisioning.' *Global Environmental Change*, Volume 69, 102287.

Walker, A. (1983). *In Search of Our Mothers' Gardens: Womanist Prose*. San Diego: Harcourt Brace Jovanovich.

Notes

1 EEB and WECF, 2021, p. 46.
2 Ibid.
3 Ibid., p.41-42.
4 Arendt, 1958, p. 6.
5 Roy, 2020
6 IPBES, 2019, p.xviii
7 Meadows, 1999, p.17
8 Hache, 2016
9 Ibid.
10 Hache, 2016 and Purtschert, 2020.
11 Hache, 2016.
12 Shiva, 1988.
13 Shiva & Bandyophadhay, 1986, p.134 and Shiva, 1988.
14 Shiva, 1988.
15 Shiva & Bandyophadhay, 1986, p.136.
16 Ibid.
17 Ibid., p.137.
18 Ibid., p.140.
19 Shiva & Bandhyophadhay, 1986, p.140 and Shiva 1988, p.67-72.
20 Mies & Shiva, 2014.
21 Hunnicutt, 2020

[22] Hache, 2016.
[23] Phillips, 2019.
[24] Ibid.
[25] Donath, 2000; Mellor, 1997, 2009; Waring, 1988 in Phillips, 2016, p.1152.
[26] Mellor, 1997 in Phillips, 2016, p.1152.
[27] Ibid.
[28] Phillips, 2016.
[29] Mies and Shiva, 2014.
[30] Ibid., p.xx-xxi.
[31] Stewart Brand in Mies & Shiva, 2014, p.xviii.
[32] Holemans, 2016, p.135.
[33] Merchant, 1980.
[34] Ibid., p.228.
[35] Following Bruno Latour (2017, p.11), climate is understood here as 'the relations between human beings and the material conditions of their lives'.
[36] This analysis has been taken from Holemans, 2016, p.136.
[37] Marçal, 2015 in Holemans, 2016, p.136.
[38] Hache, 2016.
[39] Ibid.
[40] Plumwood, 1997, p.42.
[41] See Plumwood, 1997, Chapter 2: Dualism: the logic of colonisation.
[42] https://www.denktankminerva.be/analyse/2018/2/28/vrouwen-in-deeltijdwerk-dwang-of-keuze
[43] De Beauvoir, 1965, p.8 in Plumwood, 1997, p.52.
[44] See Shiva, 1993.

45 hooks, 1989, p. 22.
46 Crenshaw, 1986.
47 Misiedjan, 2021.
48 Crenshaw, 2020.
49 Sturgeon, 1997, p.259-260.
50 Walker, 1983, p. xi.
51 Harris, 2016, p.5.
52 Harris, 2016, p.6.
53 Inspired by Rico, 2017 and Zoboi, 2017.
54 Villanueva, 2021, p.151.
55 Tutu, 2013.
56 Shiva, 2017.
57 Mies & Shiva, 2014, p.xxi.
58 Ibid.
59 See Humankind: A Hopeful History by Rutger Bregman (Bloomsbury 2020A).
60 Meadows, 1999.
61 Simard, 2021, p. 283
62 Puig de la Bellacasa, 2017, p.33.
63 Marçal, 2015, p.115.
64 de Wit, 2019.
65 See, amongst others, Holemans, 2016 and 2020.
66 Peeters, J. in Holemans, 2020.
67 See the Ferris Jabr articles 'The Social Life of Forests' (*The New York Times Magazine*, 2 December 2020) and 'The Secret Life of Plants' (*New Scientist*, 26 March 2021).
68 Https://www.waerbeke.be/columns/columnisten/jan-mertens/260-destilte-in-de-storm.
69 https://www.theguardian.com/environment/2019/

jan/25/our-house-is-on-fire-greta-thunberg16-urges-leaders-to-act-on-climate.

70 See https://bodhitv.nl/sterke-boeddhistische-vrouwen-joanna-macy/

71 In Burgers L., et al., 2020.

72 Schinkel, p.183.

73 Leopold, 1949, p.xix.

74 Fisher & Tronto, 1990, p. 40.

75 These three dimensions are highlighted by Puig de la Bellacasa, 2017.

76 Ibid.

77 Descola, 2021.

78 Joan Tronto, quoted in Peeters, 2021, p. 96 and Tronto, 2017.

79 See, for example, Holemans, 2021.

80 See https://www.dewereldmorgen.be/artikel/2021/08/19/berlijn-haalt359-000-handtekeningen-voor-referendum-over-onteigening-grote-immobilienbedrijven.

81 This brief account does not do justice to Max-Neef's ingenious perspective, which includes the matrix of needs and satisfiers. See Max-Neef, 1991.

82 Power, 2004, cited in Peeters, 2021, p.91-105.

83 Vogel et al., 2021.

84 Hickel, 2021, p.156.

85 Ibid.

86 Hickel 2021, p. 159.

87 Ibidem, p.163-4

88 Mbembe, 2016.

89 Mbembe, cited in De Walsche, 2021, p.65-74. See also Mbembe, 2016 and https://www.uantwerpen.be/en/centres/usos/webinars-masterclasses/debating-development/edition-2020--decolo/mbembe

90 See, amongst others, https://www.theafricareport.com/32162/when-haitipaid-france-for-freedom-the-greatest-heist-in-history/ and https://www.opendemocracy.net/en/north-africa-west-asia/haitian-revolution-spectre-tahrir-global-revolution-possible

91 For a detailed analysis of the various types of the rebound effect, see Holemans (2016).

92 See https://www.unrisd.org/unrisd/website/document.nsf/(httpPublications)/2D51D21D694A94D4802586A1004D18FC

Oikos

Think ahead

© Dirk Holemans, Marie-Monique Franssen, Philsan Osman
SKRIBIS is het publicatieplatform van drukkerij Mirto Print.
Publicaties bij skribis worden uitgebracht in eigen beheer.

SKRIBIS – Mirto Print cv erkend als so
Industriepark-Drongen 21
9031 Gent

Tel. 09 244 72 68
info@skribis.be
www.skribis.be

Cover: Luna Vermeire
Lay-out: www.intertext.be
GEF project coordination: Sien Hasker

Dirk Holemans, Marie-Monique Franssen, Philsan Osman
Dare to Care. Ecofeminism as a source of inspiration
Gent, 2022, 108 p.

ISBN 978 94 644 4526 8
D/2022/3988/28
NUR 740

*No part of this book may be reproduced in any form,
by print, mimeograph, film or any other means without
permission in writing from the publisher*